I0466994

LONG COVID LIFESTYLE BIBLE

Insights and Management of Long COVID

George R. Miller

COPYRIGHT

TABLE OF CONTENT

INTRODUCTION

The COVID-19 pandemic has left an indelible mark on the world, altering lives in ways unimaginable just a few years ago. While the acute phase of the virus has garnered much attention, a significant number of individuals continue to grapple with lingering symptoms long after their initial recovery. These individuals, known as COVID-19 long haulers, face a myriad of challenges that extend far beyond the acute illness. This book aims to shed light on the complexities of long COVID, offering detailed insights into its causes, symptoms, and management strategies. By weaving together scientific research, clinical expertise, and personal narratives, we hope to provide a comprehensive resource for patients, caregivers, and healthcare professionals. Our goal is to empower readers with knowledge, fostering a deeper understanding and more effective support for those affected by this enduring condition.

Overview of COVID-19

COVID-19, caused by the novel coronavirus SARS-CoV-2, emerged in late 2019 and rapidly spread worldwide, resulting in an unprecedented global pandemic. Originating in Wuhan, China, the virus is primarily transmitted through respiratory droplets, with airborne and surface transmission also contributing to its spread. COVID-19's impact has been profound, affecting every aspect of life, from healthcare and economies to social interactions and daily routines.

The virus manifests in a range of symptoms, from mild respiratory issues to severe pneumonia and multi-organ failure. Common symptoms include fever, cough, and shortness of breath, but the disease can also lead to loss of taste or smell, fatigue, and gastrointestinal issues. While many people recover without needing extensive medical care, COVID-19 can be fatal, particularly for older adults and those with underlying health conditions.

Global efforts to combat the virus have included the development and distribution of vaccines, implementation of public health measures such as social distancing and mask-wearing, and ongoing research into treatments and preventive strategies. Despite these efforts, new variants continue to challenge containment and management efforts, highlighting the need for continued vigilance and adaptation.

The pandemic has also exposed and exacerbated existing inequalities, disproportionately affecting marginalized communities. As the world navigates the ongoing challenges of COVID-19, understanding its multifaceted impact remains crucial for developing effective responses and fostering resilience in the face of future public health crises.

Definition and Significance of Long COVID

Long COVID, also known as post-acute sequelae of SARS-CoV-2 infection (PASC), refers to the condition where individuals continue to experience a wide range of symptoms for weeks or months after the acute phase of a COVID-19 infection has resolved. This syndrome can affect anyone who has had COVID-19, regardless of the severity of their initial illness, including those who were asymptomatic.

Symptoms of long COVID are diverse and can impact multiple organ systems. Commonly reported symptoms include persistent fatigue, shortness of breath, chest pain, cognitive difficulties (often referred to as "brain fog"), sleep disturbances, joint and muscle pain, and depression or anxiety. The variability and persistence of these symptoms can significantly affect daily functioning and quality of life, making long COVID a substantial public health concern.

The significance of long COVID lies in its widespread impact and the challenges it presents to healthcare systems. As millions globally have contracted COVID-19, a significant proportion may suffer from long-term consequences, placing a considerable burden on healthcare resources and services. Additionally, the economic implications are profound, with many long haulers unable to return to work or requiring ongoing medical care.

Understanding long COVID is crucial for developing effective treatment and management strategies, improving patient outcomes, and guiding public health policies. Ongoing research is essential to unravel the underlying mechanisms of this condition, identify risk factors, and develop targeted therapies to help those affected reclaim their health and lives.

Purpose and Structure of the Book

The purpose of this book is to provide a comprehensive and accessible resource on COVID-19 long haulers, a condition that has emerged as a significant and enduring challenge in the wake of the COVID-19 pandemic. By delving into the causes, symptoms, diagnosis, and treatment of long COVID, this book aims to equip patients, caregivers, and healthcare professionals with the knowledge needed to navigate this complex condition. It also seeks to raise awareness about the long-term impacts of COVID-19, advocating for more research, resources, and support for those affected.

The structure of this book is designed to offer a detailed exploration of long COVID from multiple perspectives. It begins with foundational chapters on understanding COVID-19 and the definition and significance of long COVID. Subsequent chapters delve into the causes and wide-ranging symptoms experienced by long haulers. The book then covers approaches to symptom management, diagnosis, and treatment, with specific chapters dedicated to the effects on the respiratory system and other bodily systems.

Recovery strategies are discussed, including both conventional medical approaches and herbal management plans. The book also examines innovative treatments, lifestyle modifications, and coping mechanisms. Personal stories and case studies are interwoven throughout to humanize the condition and provide real-world context. Concluding chapters focus on current research, future directions, and resources for patients and healthcare providers, ensuring a holistic and informed approach to long COVID.

I

Understanding COVID-19 Long Haulers

Definition and Terminology

COVID-19 long haulers, also referred to as individuals with long COVID or post-acute sequelae of SARS-CoV-2 infection (PASC), are those who experience persistent symptoms or new health issues long after the acute phase of a COVID-19 infection has resolved. This condition can affect anyone who has had COVID-19, regardless of the initial severity of their illness, including those who were asymptomatic or had mild cases.

The terminology surrounding long COVID is evolving as our understanding of the condition deepens. "Long COVID" is the most commonly used term, encompassing the wide range of symptoms that continue for weeks or months beyond the initial infection. The term "post-acute sequelae of SARS-CoV-2 infection" (PASC) is often used in medical literature to describe the prolonged effects that follow the acute phase of the infection. "Chronic COVID-19 syndrome" is another term sometimes used to emphasize the ongoing and chronic nature of the condition.

Long COVID can manifest through a diverse array of symptoms affecting multiple organ systems. Common symptoms include fatigue, shortness of breath, cognitive dysfunction (often referred to as "brain fog"), chest pain, joint and muscle pain, sleep disturbances, and psychological symptoms such as anxiety and depression. Understanding these terms and their implications is crucial for recognizing and addressing the needs of long haulers, ensuring they receive appropriate care and support.

Epidemiology and Demographics

The epidemiology of long COVID reflects its widespread impact, affecting a significant portion of those who have had COVID-19. Studies suggest that approximately 10-30% of individuals who recover from the acute phase of the virus experience persistent symptoms, although this rate can vary based on demographics and the severity of initial infection. Long COVID affects people of all ages, including children and adolescents, though it appears more prevalent in adults and older populations.

Demographically, long COVID seems to disproportionately affect women more than men, with some studies indicating that women are twice as likely to experience long-term symptoms. Additionally, individuals with pre-existing health conditions, such as cardiovascular disease, diabetes, or obesity, are at higher risk of developing long COVID. Socioeconomic factors also play a role, as those from marginalized communities may face increased vulnerability due to limited access to healthcare and other resources. Understanding these epidemiological patterns is essential for targeting preventive measures and healthcare interventions effectively.

Historical Perspective on Post-Viral Syndromes

Post-viral syndromes have been recognized for centuries, manifesting as prolonged symptoms following viral infections. Historically, such conditions were known by various names and were often poorly understood. One of the earliest documented post-viral syndromes is myalgic encephalomyelitis (ME), also known as chronic fatigue syndrome (CFS), which gained attention in the mid-20th century.

ME/CFS emerged as a significant concern when clusters of patients presented with persistent fatigue and other debilitating symptoms long after an acute viral illness.

Another notable example is the post-polio syndrome (PPS), which emerged in the 1980s as polio survivors began experiencing new symptoms decades after their initial infection. PPS is characterized by progressive muscle weakness, fatigue, and pain, showing that the aftereffects of viral infections can manifest many years later.

These historical examples underscore a pattern where viral infections can lead to long-term health issues, often poorly understood at the time. They highlight the necessity for ongoing research into post-viral conditions, including long COVID. The historical context provides valuable insights into how viral infections can have enduring impacts on health, emphasizing the need for comprehensive approaches to understanding and managing long-term consequences of infectious diseases.

Personal Stories and Case Studies

Personal stories and case studies are vital for understanding the lived experience of COVID-19 long haulers. These narratives offer a humanizing perspective, illustrating the profound impact of long COVID on individuals' lives. Patients often describe a range of persistent symptoms, from debilitating fatigue and cognitive impairment to ongoing respiratory issues and mental health challenges. These personal accounts reveal the daily struggles faced by long haulers, such as difficulty returning to work, managing household responsibilities, and navigating a healthcare system that is still learning about long COVID.

Case studies provide detailed insights into specific instances of long COVID, highlighting variations in symptom severity, progression, and response to treatment. They are invaluable for identifying common patterns and unique challenges, contributing to a broader understanding of the condition. By sharing these stories, we not only validate the experiences of those affected but also emphasize the urgent need for effective treatments and support systems.

Societal and Economic Impact

The societal and economic impact of long COVID is profound and multifaceted. Long-term symptoms and health issues experienced by long haulers can significantly disrupt daily life, affecting their ability to work, care for family, and participate in social activities. This ongoing disability often leads to reduced productivity and increased reliance on social support systems, placing a strain on both individuals and families.

Economically, long COVID contributes to increased healthcare costs due to the need for ongoing medical care, rehabilitation, and management of chronic symptoms. Businesses and economies also feel the impact through lost labor and reduced workforce productivity. Additionally, the psychological burden of long COVID can lead to increased mental health challenges, further exacerbating the economic toll.

Societally, the increased prevalence of long COVID highlights disparities in healthcare access and support, emphasizing the need for comprehensive public health strategies and resources to address the long-term consequences of the pandemic.

II

Theories on the Causes of Long COVID

Long COVID, characterized by persistent symptoms after the acute phase of a SARS-CoV-2 infection, remains a complex and poorly understood condition. Several theories have been proposed to explain its causes, including viral persistence, immune system dysregulation, autonomic nervous system involvement, and microclots and blood vessel damage.

Viral Persistence suggests that remnants of the SARS-CoV-2 virus may remain in the body long after the acute infection has resolved. This theory posits that viral particles or genetic material could persist in tissues such as the gastrointestinal tract or respiratory system, continuing to stimulate the immune system and cause chronic inflammation. Studies have identified viral RNA in various body tissues post-recovery, supporting the idea that viral persistence might contribute to ongoing symptoms like fatigue and cognitive dysfunction. If residual viral particles are a significant factor, targeted antiviral therapies may become crucial for managing long COVID.

Immune System Dysregulation is another leading theory. During the acute phase of COVID-19, the immune system mounts a vigorous response, which can sometimes become excessive or misdirected. This dysregulation can result in a prolonged inflammatory state or autoimmune responses, where the immune system mistakenly attacks the body's own tissues. This ongoing inflammation and autoimmunity might explain persistent symptoms such as joint pain, chronic fatigue, and brain fog. Understanding and addressing immune system abnormalities are key to developing effective treatments for long COVID.

Autonomic Nervous System Involvement suggests that long COVID might affect the autonomic nervous system (ANS), which controls involuntary functions like heart rate and blood pressure. Disruptions in the ANS could lead to symptoms such as dizziness, palpitations, and orthostatic intolerance (difficulty standing up due to blood pressure drops). This theory is supported by the observation of conditions like postural orthostatic tachycardia syndrome (POTS) in long COVID patients. If ANS dysfunction is a significant factor, treatments aimed at regulating autonomic function may be beneficial.

Microclots and Blood Vessel Damage have also been implicated in long COVID. SARS-CoV-2 infection can induce abnormal clotting and damage to small blood vessels. The presence of microclots—tiny clots obstructing small vessels—can impair blood flow and oxygen delivery, leading to symptoms such as fatigue, pain, and cognitive issues. Vascular damage and endothelial dysfunction further exacerbate these issues by contributing to chronic inflammation and poor circulation. Addressing these vascular complications through anticoagulants or therapies targeting endothelial health might offer relief to long haulers.

Each of these theories highlights a different aspect of the complex pathology of long COVID. Continued research is essential to fully understand these mechanisms and develop effective management strategies for those affected.

Overview of Symptoms

Long COVID, or post-acute sequelae of SARS-CoV-2 infection (PASC), encompasses a broad spectrum of symptoms that persist or emerge long after the acute phase of COVID-19 has resolved. These symptoms can vary widely in type and severity, affecting multiple organ systems.

Common Symptoms include:

1. Fatigue: One of the most frequently reported symptoms, fatigue in long COVID can be profound and debilitating, significantly impacting daily activities and overall quality of life.
2. Shortness of Breath: Persistent respiratory issues, including difficulty breathing or shortness of breath, are common. This can be particularly distressing for those who had mild or asymptomatic initial infections.
3. Cognitive Dysfunction: Often referred to as "brain fog," this includes difficulties with concentration, memory, and mental clarity. It can affect work performance and daily functioning.
4. Muscle and Joint Pain: Persistent aches and pains in muscles and joints are frequently reported, resembling conditions like fibromyalgia.

Less Common Symptoms include:

1. Gastrointestinal Issues: Symptoms such as nausea, diarrhea, and abdominal pain, while less common, are still reported by some long COVID patients.

2. Skin Problems: Rashes, itching, and other dermatological issues have been observed, although they are not as prevalent as other symptoms.

3. Sleep Disturbances: Insomnia or disrupted sleep patterns can be a significant issue, contributing to overall fatigue and poor quality of life.

Severe and Rare Symptoms include:

1. Cardiovascular Issues: Severe complications such as myocarditis (inflammation of the heart muscle) and pericarditis (inflammation of the lining around the heart) can occur. These conditions may cause persistent chest pain and irregular heartbeats.

2. Neurological Problems: More severe cases can involve neurological symptoms like seizures, neuropathy, or strokes, which may have lasting effects on neurological function.

3. Organ Damage: In rare cases, long COVID can lead to significant damage to organs such as the lungs or kidneys, potentially resulting in chronic respiratory or renal issues.

The variability in symptoms and their severity underscores the complexity of long COVID, highlighting the need for personalized treatment and ongoing research to better understand and manage this condition.

Symptom Duration and Variability

Symptom duration and variability in long COVID are notable for their unpredictability and wide range. For some individuals, symptoms may persist for weeks or months, extending well beyond the initial infection period. The duration can vary greatly, with some experiencing persistent issues for over a year.

Duration: Many long COVID patients report symptoms lasting for several months after the acute phase of infection. Fatigue and cognitive difficulties are particularly enduring, sometimes lasting up to 12 months or more. The chronic nature of these symptoms can significantly affect daily functioning and quality of life.

Variability: Symptoms in long COVID can be highly variable, both in type and severity. Patients may experience a fluctuating course, with symptoms worsening and improving intermittently. Some may encounter a core set of symptoms consistently, while others may develop new issues over time. This variability can make diagnosis and management challenging, as treatment needs to be tailored to the individual's evolving condition.

This variability is influenced by several factors, including the severity of the initial infection, underlying health conditions, and individual differences in immune response and recovery. Understanding and addressing this variability is crucial for effective treatment and support for long COVID patients.

Comparison with Other Post-Viral Syndromes

Long COVID shares similarities with other post-viral syndromes, such as myalgic encephalomyelitis/chronic fatigue syndrome (ME/CFS) and post-polio syndrome (PPS), yet also exhibits distinct features.

Myalgic Encephalomyelitis/Chronic Fatigue Syndrome (ME/CFS): ME/CFS is characterized by debilitating fatigue, cognitive dysfunction, and muscle pain, mirroring many symptoms seen in long COVID. Both conditions can lead to profound impairment in daily activities and overall quality of life. However, ME/CFS typically develops following a viral infection but can also be triggered by other factors. Unlike long COVID, ME/CFS has been studied longer, with established diagnostic criteria and management approaches.

Post-Polio Syndrome (PPS): PPS occurs in polio survivors years after their initial infection, manifesting as new muscle weakness and fatigue. Similar to long COVID, PPS involves a late onset of symptoms following a previous viral illness. However, PPS is specific to polio survivors, whereas long COVID can affect anyone who has had COVID-19, regardless of the severity of the initial illness.

While these post-viral syndromes share features such as persistent fatigue and cognitive issues, long COVID's broader range of symptoms and its association with a novel virus create unique challenges in understanding and managing the condition. Ongoing research aims to elucidate the similarities and differences to improve diagnosis and treatment strategies for long COVID.

III

Symptom Management Approaches

Medical Management: Effective management of long COVID symptoms often involves a multifaceted medical approach, combining medications, treatments, and lifestyle adjustments.

Medications and Treatments: Medications play a key role in alleviating specific symptoms of long COVID. For instance, anti-inflammatory drugs, such as corticosteroids, may help manage persistent inflammation. Pain relievers and muscle relaxants can address joint and muscle pain. Respiratory symptoms may be treated with bronchodilators or other pulmonary therapies. Antidepressants or anti-anxiety medications might be prescribed to address mental health challenges such as depression or anxiety, which are common among long COVID patients. Treatment plans are typically tailored to individual symptom profiles, and ongoing adjustments are often necessary to optimize effectiveness and minimize side effects.

Off-label Drug Use: In cases where conventional treatments are inadequate, off-label drug use may be considered. Off-label prescribing involves using medications that are not specifically approved for long COVID but may offer benefits based on their known effects. For example, some patients have reported improvements with medications traditionally used for other conditions, such as antivirals or immune modulators. While off-label use can provide additional options, it comes with risks, including the potential for unanticipated side effects and interactions. It is crucial for patients to discuss these options with their healthcare providers, who can help weigh the potential benefits against the risks and monitor for adverse effects.

Overall, a personalized approach to symptom management, involving both standard and off-label treatments, is essential for effectively addressing the diverse and persistent symptoms associated with long COVID.

Physical Rehabilitation

Exercise Programs: Physical rehabilitation for long COVID often incorporates structured exercise programs tailored to individual capabilities and needs. Exercise can help alleviate symptoms such as fatigue and muscle weakness, improve cardiovascular health, and enhance overall physical function. Programs typically include aerobic activities, strength training, and flexibility exercises. Aerobic exercises, such as walking or cycling, help improve endurance and cardiovascular health. Strength training focuses on rebuilding muscle strength and stamina, which can be significantly impaired in long COVID patients. Flexibility exercises, like stretching or yoga, can enhance mobility and reduce discomfort. Exercise programs are usually designed in collaboration with healthcare providers to ensure they are safe, effective, and gradually adjusted based on patient progress.

Physiotherapy Techniques: Physiotherapy techniques are crucial for managing musculoskeletal symptoms and improving overall physical function. Techniques may include manual therapy, which involves hands-on manipulation of muscles and joints to relieve pain and improve movement. Therapeutic exercises prescribed by a physiotherapist help strengthen weak muscles, improve posture, and increase range of motion. Additionally, techniques like heat and cold therapy, as well as electrical stimulation, may be used to alleviate pain and promote healing. Physiotherapy aims to restore functional capacity and improve the quality of life for long COVID patients.

Respiratory Therapy: Respiratory therapy is essential for managing long COVID-related respiratory symptoms. This therapy involves techniques to improve lung function, enhance breathing efficiency, and reduce symptoms such as shortness of breath and chronic cough. Techniques may include breathing exercises, such as diaphragmatic breathing or pursed-lip breathing, to strengthen respiratory muscles and improve oxygenation. Additionally, respiratory therapists may use devices like nebulizers or inhalers to administer medications that help open airways and reduce inflammation. Regular respiratory therapy sessions can support lung recovery and overall respiratory health in long COVID patients.

Together, these physical rehabilitation approaches—exercise programs, physiotherapy techniques, and respiratory therapy—play a crucial role in helping long COVID patients regain functional capacity and improve their quality of life.

Mental Health Support

Psychological Counseling: Psychological counseling is a critical component of mental health support for individuals experiencing long COVID. Chronic illness can lead to or exacerbate mental health issues such as anxiety, depression, and stress. Professional counselors or therapists provide a safe space for patients to express their feelings and work through the emotional challenges associated with long COVID. Counseling helps patients develop coping strategies, improve their emotional resilience, and address any underlying psychological issues that may be affecting their well-being. Through various therapeutic techniques, counselors support patients in navigating the complexities of their condition and fostering a sense of control and hope.

Cognitive Behavioral Therapy (CBT): Cognitive Behavioral Therapy (CBT) is an evidence-based therapeutic approach that is particularly effective in managing the mental health aspects of long COVID. CBT focuses on identifying and challenging negative thought patterns and behaviors that contribute to emotional distress. By teaching patients how to reframe their thoughts, set realistic goals, and develop problem-solving skills, CBT helps them better manage symptoms of anxiety, depression, and stress. This therapy also incorporates strategies for improving daily functioning and building resilience, which are essential for coping with the ongoing challenges of long COVID.

Support Groups: Support groups offer invaluable peer support for individuals living with long COVID. These groups, whether in-person or online, provide a platform for patients to connect with others who share similar experiences. Participating in support groups helps reduce feelings of isolation and provides opportunities for sharing coping strategies and emotional support. Group settings also foster a sense of community and understanding, which can be empowering and reassuring for individuals navigating the uncertainties of long COVID. Through mutual support and shared experiences, patients can gain practical advice, emotional comfort, and a sense of belonging.

Diet and Nutrition

Diet and nutrition play a crucial role in managing long COVID, as proper dietary habits can help mitigate symptoms, support overall health, and enhance recovery. Several dietary strategies, including anti-inflammatory diets, nutritional supplements, and maintaining hydration and electrolyte balance, are particularly relevant for long COVID patients.

Anti-inflammatory Diets: Chronic inflammation is a common feature of long COVID, and an anti-inflammatory diet can help reduce inflammation and support immune function. Such diets emphasize the consumption of foods rich in antioxidants and anti-inflammatory compounds. Key components include:

- Fruits and Vegetables: Rich in vitamins, minerals, and antioxidants, these foods help combat oxidative stress and inflammation. Berries, leafy greens, and cruciferous vegetables like broccoli are particularly beneficial.
- Healthy Fats: Omega-3 fatty acids, found in fatty fish (e.g., salmon), flaxseeds, and walnuts, have potent anti-inflammatory properties. Olive oil is another excellent source of healthy fats that can help reduce inflammation.
- Whole Grains: Whole grains like oats, brown rice, and quinoa provide fiber and essential nutrients, which contribute to overall health and may reduce inflammation.
- Spices and Herbs: Turmeric and ginger are known for their anti-inflammatory effects and can be easily incorporated into meals.

Nutritional Supplements: Certain supplements may help address deficiencies and support recovery. While supplements should not replace a balanced diet, they can complement nutritional needs, especially in long COVID:

- Vitamin D: Important for immune function, vitamin D deficiency is common in many individuals and may be linked to increased susceptibility to infections. Supplementation can help maintain adequate levels.

- Vitamin C and Zinc: Both play roles in supporting the immune system and may have beneficial effects in reducing inflammation and supporting recovery.

- Probiotics: Gut health can influence overall immune function. Probiotic supplements may help maintain a healthy gut microbiome, potentially improving immune responses and reducing gastrointestinal symptoms.

Hydration and Electrolyte Balance: Maintaining proper hydration and electrolyte balance is essential for overall health and can be particularly important for long COVID patients who may experience symptoms such as fatigue, dizziness, or muscle cramps. Adequate hydration supports bodily functions, including circulation and digestion, and helps prevent dehydration.

- Water: Drinking sufficient water is fundamental to maintaining hydration. Aim to consume at least eight glasses of water daily, or more if symptoms like fever or diarrhea are present.

- Electrolytes: Electrolytes like sodium, potassium, and magnesium are crucial for maintaining fluid balance and muscle function. Including electrolyte-rich foods such as bananas, avocados, and coconut water in the diet can help maintain balance, especially if there is significant fluid loss due to symptoms like sweating or gastrointestinal disturbances.

Incorporating these dietary strategies into a long COVID management plan can help alleviate symptoms, support overall health, and enhance recovery. However, dietary changes should be made in consultation with healthcare providers to ensure they align with individual health needs and conditions.

IV

Criteria for Diagnosis

Diagnosing long COVID involves a comprehensive evaluation that includes clinical assessment and a thorough review of patient history and symptom tracking.

Clinical Assessment: The diagnosis of long COVID typically starts with a detailed clinical assessment by a healthcare provider. This includes a physical examination and evaluation of persistent symptoms that continue beyond the acute phase of COVID-19, usually lasting for more than 12 weeks. Symptoms may include fatigue, breathlessness, cognitive issues, and joint pain. The assessment also involves ruling out other potential causes of the symptoms through tests and investigations, such as blood tests, imaging studies, and pulmonary function tests. This process ensures that other conditions are not contributing to the patient's ongoing symptoms.

Patient History and Symptom Tracking: A thorough patient history is critical in diagnosing long COVID. This includes reviewing the patient's initial COVID-19 infection, its severity, and the timeline of symptom onset. Symptom tracking involves documenting the duration, frequency, and intensity of symptoms over time. This tracking helps establish a pattern consistent with long COVID and differentiates it from other post-viral syndromes or chronic conditions. Accurate and detailed symptom tracking provides valuable information for diagnosis and guides appropriate management strategies.

Combining these approaches helps establish a diagnosis of long COVID and ensures a targeted and effective treatment plan.

Diagnostic Tests

Diagnostic tests are essential in evaluating long COVID, helping to confirm the diagnosis, assess the extent of organ involvement, and rule out other conditions. The primary categories of diagnostic tests for long COVID include blood tests and biomarkers, as well as imaging and functional tests.

Blood Tests and Biomarkers: Blood tests are crucial for identifying underlying inflammation, immune system abnormalities, and other potential contributors to long COVID symptoms. Commonly measured biomarkers include:

- Inflammatory Markers: Levels of markers such as C-reactive protein (CRP) and erythrocyte sedimentation rate (ESR) can indicate ongoing inflammation, which is often present in long COVID.
- Immune Function Tests: Tests assessing levels of specific immune cells or antibodies can provide insights into immune system dysregulation.
- Vitamin and Mineral Levels: Evaluating deficiencies or imbalances in vitamins (e.g., vitamin D) and minerals (e.g., zinc) can help identify nutritional deficiencies that may contribute to symptoms.

Imaging and Functional Tests: Imaging and functional tests are used to evaluate organ function and detect potential damage caused by long COVID:

- Chest X-rays and CT Scans: These imaging modalities assess lung function and identify structural changes or damage, such as pulmonary fibrosis or residual inflammation. They are essential for evaluating respiratory symptoms and guiding treatment.

- Pulmonary Function Tests (PFTs): PFTs measure lung capacity and airflow, helping to assess the impact of long COVID on respiratory function.
- Cardiac Imaging: Echocardiograms or MRIs can be used to evaluate heart function and detect conditions like myocarditis, which may be related to long COVID symptoms.

Together, these diagnostic tests provide a comprehensive understanding of the impact of long COVID on the body, guiding treatment decisions and management strategies.

Treatment Protocols

Standard Treatment Guidelines: The management of long COVID often involves a multidisciplinary approach based on symptom relief and overall well-being. Standard treatment protocols are designed to address the diverse range of symptoms and improve quality of life:

- Symptom Management: Treatment typically includes medications for specific symptoms such as fatigue, pain, and respiratory issues. For example, analgesics or anti-inflammatory drugs may be used to alleviate muscle and joint pain, while bronchodilators and inhaled corticosteroids can manage persistent respiratory symptoms.

- Rehabilitation Therapies: Physical therapy and rehabilitation are key components of treatment, focusing on improving physical function and endurance. Exercise programs are tailored to individual tolerance levels to help restore strength and stamina.

- Mental Health Support: Psychological counseling and cognitive behavioral therapy are employed to address anxiety, depression, and cognitive impairments. Support groups also provide valuable emotional support and practical advice for coping with long COVID.

Emerging and Experimental Therapies: As research into long COVID progresses, several emerging and experimental therapies are being explored:

- Novel Medications: New medications targeting specific pathways involved in long COVID, such as anti-inflammatory agents or immune-modulating drugs, are under investigation. These treatments aim to address underlying mechanisms of the condition and provide more effective symptom relief.

- Immune System Modulation: Therapies that modify immune responses, including monoclonal antibodies and other immunotherapies, are being studied for their potential to manage persistent inflammation and immune dysregulation.

- Regenerative Medicine: Research into regenerative therapies, such as stem cell treatments, aims to repair or regenerate damaged tissues and organs affected by long COVID. These therapies are in experimental stages and require further validation.

Overall, treatment protocols for long COVID are evolving, incorporating both established guidelines and innovative approaches to provide comprehensive care tailored to individual needs. Ongoing research and clinical trials will continue to shape the future of long COVID management.

Specialized Clinics

Role and Function of Long COVID Clinics: Long COVID clinics are specialized centers dedicated to the diagnosis, treatment, and management of long COVID. These clinics are designed to address the complex and multifaceted nature of the condition, offering comprehensive care tailored to the unique needs of each patient. The primary roles of long COVID clinics include providing accurate diagnoses, developing personalized treatment plans, and offering ongoing support for symptom management and recovery.

Multidisciplinary Approach: One of the key strengths of long COVID clinics is their multidisciplinary approach. These clinics typically bring together a diverse team of healthcare professionals, including:

- Pulmonologists: Specialists who focus on respiratory issues, such as persistent cough or breathlessness, and conduct pulmonary function tests.
- Cardiologists: Experts in managing cardiovascular symptoms and evaluating heart function through imaging and other diagnostic tools.
- Neurologists: Professionals who address cognitive and neurological symptoms, including memory problems and brain fog.
- Rehabilitation Specialists: Physical therapists and occupational therapists who develop and implement exercise and rehabilitation programs to improve physical function and manage fatigue.
- Psychologists/Psychiatrists: Mental health professionals who provide counseling, cognitive behavioral therapy, and support for anxiety, depression, and other psychological aspects of long COVID.

This integrated approach ensures that all aspects of the patient's condition are addressed, from physical symptoms to psychological well-being. Long COVID clinics also offer continuity of care, with regular follow-ups and adjustments to treatment plans based on patient progress and evolving symptoms. By combining expertise across various medical disciplines, long COVID clinics aim to provide holistic and effective management for patients navigating the challenges of long COVID.

V

Respiratory Symptoms

Shortness of Breath: One of the most common respiratory symptoms reported by long COVID patients is shortness of breath, or dyspnea. This sensation of difficulty or discomfort in breathing can vary in intensity, from mild to severe. Shortness of breath may occur during physical activity or even at rest. It is often linked to inflammation or damage to the lungs and airways caused by the initial COVID-19 infection. Pulmonary function tests can assess the severity of this symptom and help in managing it. Treatment strategies may include the use of bronchodilators, inhaled corticosteroids, and pulmonary rehabilitation exercises to improve lung function and breathing capacity.

Chronic Cough: A persistent, chronic cough is another prevalent respiratory issue among long COVID patients. This cough may be dry or productive and can linger for weeks or months after the acute phase of COVID-19. It can be caused by ongoing inflammation of the airways, residual viral infection, or damage to the respiratory tract.

Managing a chronic cough often involves identifying and treating underlying causes, which may include using cough suppressants, expectorants to clear mucus, or anti-inflammatory medications to reduce airway inflammation. In some cases, referral to a pulmonologist or an otolaryngologist (ENT specialist) may be necessary for further evaluation and treatment.

Chest Pain: Chest pain associated with long COVID can range from a mild, aching discomfort to sharp, severe pain. It may be related to inflammation of the pleura (the lining around the lungs) or other structures in the chest. While chest pain can be concerning and may require urgent evaluation to rule out serious conditions such as myocarditis or pulmonary embolism, it is often attributed to post-viral inflammation or muscle strain from persistent coughing. Treatment may include analgesics for pain relief, anti-inflammatory medications, and breathing exercises to improve lung function and reduce discomfort.

Overall, managing respiratory symptoms in long COVID requires a comprehensive approach that includes pharmacological treatments, lifestyle modifications, and specialized therapies to address the underlying causes and improve quality of life.

Lung Function Tests

Lung function tests are essential for assessing respiratory health in long COVID patients, helping to evaluate the extent of lung damage and guide appropriate treatment strategies. Key tests include spirometry, pulse oximetry, and imaging studies such as CT scans and X-rays.

Spirometry: Spirometry is a fundamental pulmonary function test that measures various aspects of lung function, including forced vital capacity (FVC) and forced expiratory volume in one second (FEV1). FVC represents the total amount of air a person can exhale after a full inhalation, while FEV1 measures the amount of air expelled in the first second of the exhalation. Reduced FEV1/FVC ratio may indicate obstructive lung diseases, such as asthma or chronic obstructive pulmonary disease (COPD), which can be a consequence of severe COVID-19. Spirometry helps identify these abnormalities and track changes in lung function over time, guiding treatment decisions and evaluating the effectiveness of interventions.

Pulse Oximetry: Pulse oximetry is a non-invasive test that measures the oxygen saturation level in the blood. It involves placing a small sensor on a finger or earlobe to assess how effectively oxygen is being transported from the lungs to the rest of the body. Normal oxygen saturation levels are typically between 95% and 100%. Lower levels may indicate issues with lung function or oxygen exchange, which are common in long COVID patients. Pulse oximetry provides real-time data on a patient's oxygen levels, which is useful for monitoring and managing respiratory symptoms.

Imaging Studies (CT, X-ray): Imaging studies, including chest X-rays and CT scans, are used to visualize the structure of the lungs and detect abnormalities. A chest X-ray can identify issues such as lung inflammation, fluid accumulation, or structural changes. A CT scan provides more detailed images, allowing for the assessment of subtle changes such as ground-glass opacities or pulmonary fibrosis, which may persist after the acute phase of COVID-19. These imaging studies help in diagnosing complications, evaluating the extent of lung damage, and monitoring recovery over time.

Together, these lung function tests provide a comprehensive evaluation of respiratory health, enabling clinicians to develop targeted treatment plans and track progress in long COVID patients.

Long-Term Respiratory Impact

Post-Viral Bronchitis: Long COVID can lead to post-viral bronchitis, a condition characterized by persistent inflammation of the bronchial tubes following an initial viral infection. Patients may experience ongoing cough, mucus production, and wheezing. This condition arises from residual inflammation or damage to the airways caused by COVID-19. Management typically involves medications to reduce inflammation and symptoms, such as corticosteroids and bronchodilators. Ensuring proper hydration and using expectorants may also help alleviate mucus buildup.

Interstitial Lung Disease (ILD): Interstitial lung disease is a serious long-term consequence of severe COVID-19. It involves inflammation and scarring of the lung tissue, leading to impaired lung function and progressive respiratory symptoms. Patients with ILD may experience persistent shortness of breath, dry cough, and reduced exercise tolerance. Diagnosing ILD involves imaging studies, such as high-resolution CT scans, which can reveal characteristic patterns of lung damage. Treatment options include anti-fibrotic medications to slow disease progression and manage symptoms, alongside supportive care.

Pulmonary Rehabilitation: Pulmonary rehabilitation is a comprehensive program designed to improve respiratory function and overall quality of life for long COVID patients. It includes exercise training to enhance endurance and strength, breathing techniques to optimize lung function, and education on managing respiratory symptoms. The program is tailored to individual needs and may involve physical therapists, respiratory therapists, and dietitians. Pulmonary rehabilitation helps patients regain physical capacity, manage symptoms more effectively, and improve overall well-being, addressing both physical and psychological aspects of recovery.

These long-term respiratory impacts highlight the importance of ongoing management and supportive care for long COVID patients, focusing on both symptomatic relief and functional improvement.

VI

Effects on the Body

Effects on the Body: Cardiovascular System

Long COVID can significantly impact the cardiovascular system, leading to a range of symptoms and conditions that affect heart function and overall circulatory health. Key cardiovascular effects include heart palpitations, chest pain, and Postural Orthostatic Tachycardia Syndrome (POTS).

Heart Palpitations: Heart palpitations, characterized by an irregular or rapid heartbeat, are a common symptom reported by long COVID patients. These sensations can range from mild fluttering to more pronounced and distressing feelings of the heart racing or pounding. Palpitations may be due to inflammation or damage to the heart muscle or autonomic nervous system dysregulation caused by the viral infection. In some cases, underlying arrhythmias or abnormalities in heart rhythm may also be contributing factors.

Managing palpitations often involves lifestyle modifications, stress management, and, if necessary, medications to stabilize heart rhythm and reduce symptoms.

Chest Pain: Persistent chest pain is another cardiovascular symptom observed in long COVID patients. The pain can vary from sharp or stabbing to dull or aching and may be related to inflammation of the pericardium (the heart's lining) or the result of ongoing stress on the heart. Chest pain can also be linked to other complications, such as myocarditis (inflammation of the heart muscle). Evaluating chest pain involves ruling out serious conditions like myocardial infarction (heart attack) through diagnostic tests such as electrocardiograms (ECGs) and cardiac imaging. Treatment typically focuses on addressing the underlying cause of the pain and providing symptomatic relief.

Postural Orthostatic Tachycardia Syndrome (POTS): POTS is a condition characterized by a significant increase in heart rate upon standing up, often accompanied by symptoms like dizziness, fatigue, and palpitations. It is thought to result from dysregulation of the autonomic nervous system, which may be triggered or exacerbated by COVID-19. Patients with POTS experience a rapid heart rate (tachycardia) when moving from a lying to a standing position, which can lead to symptoms of lightheadedness and fainting. Management includes lifestyle changes such as increased fluid and salt intake, physical conditioning exercises, and medications to regulate heart rate and blood pressure.

Overall, addressing these cardiovascular effects in long COVID requires a comprehensive approach, including diagnostic evaluation, symptom management, and interdisciplinary care to optimize cardiovascular health and support overall recovery.

Neurological Impact

Long COVID can have significant effects on the neurological system, leading to a range of symptoms that affect cognitive function, pain perception, and peripheral nerves. Key neurological impacts include brain fog and cognitive dysfunction, headaches and migraines, and neuropathy.

Brain Fog and Cognitive Dysfunction: Brain fog is a prevalent symptom among long COVID patients, characterized by difficulties with concentration, memory, and overall cognitive function. Patients often report feeling mentally sluggish, with impaired ability to focus or process information. This cognitive dysfunction can significantly affect daily activities and overall quality of life. The underlying mechanisms may involve persistent inflammation, neuroinflammation, or disruption in brain function due to the viral infection. Management strategies include cognitive rehabilitation exercises, mental stimulation activities, and ensuring adequate rest and stress management to support cognitive health.

Headaches and Migraines: Persistent headaches and migraines are common among long COVID patients. These headaches can range from tension-type headaches to more severe, disabling migraines. Migraines may be accompanied by symptoms such as nausea, sensitivity to light, and visual disturbances. The exact cause of these headaches is not fully understood, but they may be related to ongoing inflammation, changes in brain chemistry, or disruptions in blood flow. Treatment often involves a combination of medications, including analgesics and triptans for acute relief, as well as preventive measures such as lifestyle modifications, stress management techniques, and dietary adjustments to reduce headache frequency and severity.

Neuropathy: Neuropathy, or nerve damage, can manifest as tingling, numbness, or pain in the extremities. Long COVID patients may experience peripheral neuropathy due to the direct effects of the virus on nerve tissues or as a consequence of inflammatory processes. This condition can impact the quality of life by causing discomfort and impairing sensory or motor functions. Management includes medications to alleviate pain and discomfort, physical therapy to maintain mobility, and addressing any underlying inflammatory or metabolic issues that may contribute to nerve damage.

Overall, addressing the neurological impacts of long COVID involves a multidisciplinary approach to manage symptoms, support cognitive function, and enhance overall neurological health.

Musculoskeletal System

Long COVID can profoundly affect the musculoskeletal system, leading to symptoms such as joint pain and swelling, as well as muscle aches and weakness. These symptoms can significantly impact daily activities and overall quality of life.

Joint Pain and Swelling: Joint pain and swelling are common complaints among long COVID patients, often resulting from inflammation in the joints. This inflammation may be a direct consequence of the viral infection or an immune response triggered by COVID-19. Patients may experience pain, stiffness, and swelling in various joints, including knees, wrists, and elbows. Management typically involves anti-inflammatory medications, such as nonsteroidal anti-inflammatory drugs (NSAIDs), to reduce pain and swelling. In addition, physical therapy may be recommended to maintain joint function and prevent further damage. Joint protection strategies and ergonomic adjustments can also help minimize stress on affected joints.

Muscle Aches and Weakness: Muscle aches, or myalgia, and weakness are frequently reported by individuals with long COVID. These symptoms may arise from muscle inflammation or prolonged inactivity during the acute phase of the illness. Muscle weakness can impact physical function and endurance, making it challenging to perform everyday tasks. Treatment strategies for muscle aches and weakness include a combination of rest, gentle stretching, and progressive strengthening exercises. Physical therapy plays a crucial role in rehabilitating affected muscles, improving strength, and enhancing overall physical fitness. Additionally, maintaining adequate nutrition and hydration is important for muscle health and recovery.

Incorporating these management strategies can help alleviate musculoskeletal symptoms and support recovery for long COVID patients. A comprehensive approach, including medication, physical therapy, and lifestyle modifications, is essential for effective symptom management and improving overall quality of life.

Other Systems

Gastrointestinal Symptoms: Long COVID can impact the gastrointestinal (GI) system, leading to a variety of symptoms such as abdominal pain, diarrhea, nausea, and loss of appetite. These symptoms may persist long after the initial infection and can significantly affect daily functioning. The underlying causes may include ongoing inflammation, alterations in gut microbiota, or direct viral effects on the GI tract. Management strategies involve dietary modifications, such as eating small, frequent meals and avoiding irritants like spicy foods or caffeine. Probiotics may help restore gut balance, and medications such as anti-nausea agents or antidiarrheals can provide symptom relief. Consulting a gastroenterologist for persistent or severe symptoms is recommended to rule out other underlying conditions.

Dermatological Manifestations: Dermatological issues are also reported among long COVID patients. These may include skin rashes, itchiness, and changes in skin texture or color. Common conditions observed include COVID toes, characterized by swelling and discoloration of the toes, and other rashes resembling hives or eczema.

The skin manifestations may result from inflammatory responses or direct effects of the virus on the skin. Treatment typically involves topical medications to manage symptoms, such as corticosteroids for rashes or antihistamines for itching. Consulting a dermatologist can help in diagnosing and managing these skin conditions effectively.

Reproductive Health Impacts: Long COVID may also affect reproductive health. Women may experience menstrual irregularities, such as changes in cycle length or flow, while men might face sexual dysfunction or reduced libido. These symptoms could be due to hormonal imbalances or stress related to the illness. Addressing reproductive health concerns involves a multidisciplinary approach, including gynecological or urological assessments, hormonal evaluations, and counseling to manage stress and emotional impacts. Collaborative care with specialists can help address these issues and support overall reproductive health and well-being.

Managing the effects of long COVID on these various systems requires a holistic approach to ensure comprehensive care and improve quality of life.

VII

Means of Recovery

Recovery Timeline: The timeline for recovery from long COVID can vary widely among individuals, reflecting the complex nature of the condition and its impact on different body systems. Recovery typically occurs in phases, with each phase characterized by gradual improvement in symptoms and overall health.

Phases of Recovery:

1. Acute Phase: This initial phase may last several weeks to months and is marked by persistent symptoms and a significant impact on daily functioning. During this period, the focus is on symptom management and stabilization.

2. Subacute Phase: In this phase, symptoms begin to improve, and patients may experience gradual relief from the more debilitating aspects of long COVID. Rehabilitation efforts, including physical therapy and mental health support, are often emphasized.

3. Chronic Phase: For some individuals, recovery extends into the chronic phase, where symptoms persist at a lower intensity. Ongoing

management and support are crucial to maintaining quality of life and addressing any lingering issues.

Factors Influencing Recovery Time: Several factors can influence the duration and progression of recovery. These include the severity of the initial COVID-19 infection, the presence of pre-existing health conditions, individual variations in immune response, and the effectiveness of treatment and rehabilitation efforts. Lifestyle factors such as nutrition, physical activity, and stress management also play a significant role in shaping recovery outcomes. Comprehensive and individualized care plans can support a more efficient and sustained recovery process.

Rehabilitation Programs

Structured Exercise Plans: Structured exercise plans are crucial components of rehabilitation for long COVID patients, aimed at restoring physical function and endurance. These plans are tailored to the individual's current fitness level and symptoms, ensuring a gradual and safe return to physical activity. Exercise regimens often include a mix of aerobic exercises, strength training, and flexibility exercises. Aerobic exercises, such as walking, cycling, or swimming, help improve cardiovascular fitness and stamina. Strength training exercises target muscle groups affected by weakness, while flexibility exercises enhance joint mobility and reduce stiffness. Exercise programs are typically designed to start with low-intensity activities and progressively increase in intensity as tolerated. Regular assessment by a physical therapist helps adjust the program based on progress and symptom changes, ensuring that the exercise plan remains effective and safe.

Occupational Therapy: Occupational therapy plays a significant role in the rehabilitation of long COVID patients, focusing on improving the ability to perform daily activities and enhancing overall quality of life. Occupational therapists assess how symptoms impact daily functions and develop personalized strategies to address these challenges. This may include adaptive techniques for tasks such as cooking, cleaning, and personal care, as well as recommendations for ergonomic adjustments to reduce strain during activities. Therapists also provide guidance on energy conservation techniques to manage fatigue and improve task efficiency. Cognitive rehabilitation is another key aspect, helping patients with cognitive impairments to regain skills and develop coping strategies for managing memory and concentration issues. By addressing both physical and cognitive challenges, occupational therapy supports patients in achieving greater independence and improving their functional capacity in daily life.

Together, structured exercise plans and occupational therapy provide a comprehensive approach to rehabilitation, facilitating recovery and enhancing the overall well-being of long COVID patients.

Self-Care Strategies

Energy Conservation Techniques: Energy conservation techniques are essential for long COVID patients who experience persistent fatigue. These strategies help manage energy levels throughout the day by balancing activity with rest. Techniques include prioritizing tasks, breaking them into smaller, more manageable steps, and using assistive devices or modifications to reduce physical strain. Patients are encouraged to recognize their energy limits and plan activities around periods of higher energy. Employing rest breaks and avoiding overexertion can help prevent fatigue from becoming overwhelming.

Pacing and Activity Management: Pacing is a crucial strategy for managing activity levels and avoiding exacerbation of symptoms. It involves setting realistic goals, scheduling rest periods between activities, and monitoring symptoms to avoid pushing beyond one's limits. Patients should create a balanced daily routine that includes time for both activity and rest, ensuring they do not engage in strenuous tasks when their energy levels are low. Keeping a symptom diary can help track patterns and adjust activity levels accordingly. Gradual increases in activity can help build endurance without triggering setbacks.

Sleep Hygiene: Proper sleep hygiene is vital for overall health and recovery in long COVID patients. Establishing a consistent sleep schedule, creating a relaxing bedtime routine, and maintaining a comfortable sleep environment are key practices. This includes limiting exposure to screens before bedtime, avoiding stimulants like caffeine in the evening, and ensuring a dark, quiet, and cool sleeping area. Good sleep hygiene promotes restorative sleep, which is essential for physical and mental recovery. Addressing sleep disturbances, such as insomnia or sleep apnea, with the help of healthcare professionals can further enhance overall well-being.

Implementing these self-care strategies can significantly improve the quality of life for long COVID patients by managing fatigue, balancing activities, and ensuring adequate rest.

VIII

Herbal Management Plan

Overview of Herbal Medicine: Herbal medicine involves using plant-based substances for therapeutic purposes to support health and treat various conditions. This approach has been utilized for thousands of years across different cultures and remains an important aspect of traditional medicine.

History and Principles: The use of herbal remedies dates back to ancient civilizations, including those in China, India, and Egypt. Early herbalists relied on observations of plant properties and their effects on health, developing extensive pharmacopoeias that are still referenced today. Herbal medicine operates on principles such as balance and harmony, aiming to restore the body's natural equilibrium. Traditional practices often involve a holistic view of health, considering physical, emotional, and spiritual well-being. The formulation of herbal treatments typically includes single herbs or combinations designed to address specific health issues, such as inflammation or immune support.

Role in Modern Healthcare: In contemporary healthcare, herbal medicine is increasingly recognized for its potential benefits in managing chronic conditions, including long COVID. Modern research has validated some traditional uses of herbs and explored their mechanisms of action. Herbs such as turmeric, ginger, and echinacea have been studied for their anti-inflammatory, antioxidant, and immune-supporting properties. Integration of herbal medicine into mainstream healthcare involves careful consideration of efficacy, safety, and potential interactions with conventional treatments. Herbal remedies are often used as complementary treatments alongside conventional therapies to enhance overall well-being and support recovery. Collaboration between healthcare providers and herbalists ensures that these treatments are used safely and effectively within a comprehensive care plan.

Overall, herbal medicine offers valuable options for managing long COVID symptoms and promoting health, provided it is used judiciously and in conjunction with conventional medical approaches.

Common Herbal Remedies for Long COVID

Anti-inflammatory Herbs: Chronic inflammation is a key feature of long COVID, making anti-inflammatory herbs particularly valuable. Turmeric, with its active compound curcumin, is renowned for its potent anti-inflammatory and antioxidant properties. It helps reduce inflammation and oxidative stress, potentially alleviating symptoms associated with long COVID. Ginger is another effective anti-inflammatory herb that can help with joint pain and muscle aches. It contains compounds like gingerol that inhibit inflammatory pathways, providing relief from persistent inflammatory symptoms.

Immune-Modulating Herbs: Immune-modulating herbs help balance and support the immune system, which can be crucial for long COVID patients experiencing immune dysregulation. Echinacea is well-known for its ability to enhance immune function and combat infections. It stimulates the activity of white blood cells and supports overall immune health. Astragalus is another herb with immune-modulating properties, often used in traditional medicine to strengthen the immune system and improve resistance to infections. Both herbs can be beneficial in managing symptoms and supporting recovery by promoting a balanced immune response.

Adaptogenic Herbs: Adaptogenic herbs help the body cope with stress and restore balance, which can be particularly useful for long COVID patients experiencing fatigue and cognitive dysfunction.

Ashwagandha is a prominent adaptogen that helps reduce stress, improve energy levels, and support mental clarity. Rhodiola rosea is another adaptogen that enhances physical endurance, reduces fatigue, and improves cognitive function. These herbs support the body's ability to adapt to stressors and promote overall resilience, aiding in the recovery process.

Incorporating these herbal remedies into a comprehensive management plan for long COVID can help address various symptoms and support overall well-being, provided they are used under professional guidance and in conjunction with conventional treatments.

Evidence-Based Herbal Treatments

Scientific Studies and Clinical Trials: Evidence-based herbal treatments rely on rigorous scientific research to validate their efficacy and safety. Clinical trials and studies are essential for understanding how herbal remedies work and their impact on specific conditions. For instance, turmeric's active compound, curcumin, has been extensively studied for its anti-inflammatory and antioxidant properties, with numerous trials demonstrating its potential benefits in reducing inflammation and supporting overall health. Similarly, research on ginger has shown its effectiveness in alleviating nausea and reducing muscle pain. Evidence from such studies provides a foundation for incorporating these herbs into treatment plans, ensuring they are used based on reliable data.

Case Reports and Anecdotal Evidence: In addition to scientific studies, case reports and anecdotal evidence offer insights into the real-world application of herbal treatments. Case reports document individual experiences with herbal remedies, highlighting potential benefits and side effects observed in clinical settings. While anecdotal evidence is less rigorous than scientific studies, it can provide valuable insights into how herbs may work for certain individuals and help identify trends or patterns in their effectiveness. For example, many long COVID patients have reported improvements in symptoms with the use of immune-modulating herbs like echinacea, although such reports should be considered alongside more formal research.

Combining evidence from scientific studies with clinical experiences helps create a well-rounded understanding of herbal treatments, supporting their use in managing long COVID while ensuring safety and efficacy.

Integrative Medicine

Combining Herbal and Conventional Treatments: Integrative medicine focuses on combining conventional medical approaches with complementary therapies, such as herbal treatments, to enhance overall patient care. For long COVID patients, integrating herbal remedies with conventional treatments can provide a holistic approach to managing symptoms and supporting recovery. For instance, anti-inflammatory herbs like turmeric may be used alongside conventional anti-inflammatory medications to improve symptom control and potentially reduce reliance on pharmaceuticals. Immune-modulating herbs such as echinacea can complement standard treatments aimed at boosting immune function. By blending these approaches, patients benefit from a broader range of therapeutic options, addressing symptoms from multiple angles.

Safety and Efficacy Considerations: When integrating herbal and conventional treatments, safety and efficacy are paramount. It is essential to consider potential interactions between herbal remedies and prescription medications. Some herbs can affect drug metabolism or amplify side effects, necessitating careful monitoring and consultation with healthcare providers. For example, herbs like garlic and ginkgo biloba may influence blood clotting, which could interact with anticoagulant medications. Additionally, ensuring that herbal treatments are supported by scientific evidence helps verify their effectiveness and safety. Healthcare professionals should guide the selection and use of herbal remedies to avoid adverse effects and ensure that they complement rather than conflict with conventional treatments. This integrative approach aims to enhance patient outcomes while maintaining a focus on safety and informed decision-making.

Overall, integrative medicine offers a comprehensive strategy for managing long COVID, merging the strengths of herbal and conventional treatments to support recovery and improve patient well-being.

Safety and Interactions

Herb-Drug Interactions: Herb-drug interactions are a critical consideration when incorporating herbal remedies into a treatment plan, particularly for individuals taking prescription medications. Some herbs can affect the metabolism of drugs by altering liver enzyme activity, potentially leading to increased or decreased drug levels in the body. For example, St. John's Wort is known to induce liver enzymes that can reduce the effectiveness of various medications, including antidepressants and contraceptives. Similarly, herbs like ginkgo biloba and garlic can impact blood clotting, which may interfere with anticoagulant medications and increase bleeding risk. It is essential to inform healthcare providers of all herbal supplements being used to assess potential interactions and adjust treatment plans accordingly.

Precautions and Contraindications: Precautions and contraindications are crucial for ensuring the safe use of herbal remedies. Some herbs may not be suitable for individuals with specific health conditions or those who are pregnant or breastfeeding. For example, echinacea, while beneficial for immune support, may not be recommended for people with autoimmune disorders due to its immune-stimulating effects. Additionally, herbs with stimulating properties, such as ginseng, may need to be avoided by individuals with high blood pressure or heart conditions. Consulting with healthcare professionals before starting any herbal treatment is essential to identify potential contraindications and ensure that the chosen remedies do not adversely affect existing health conditions or interact with prescribed medications.

By understanding and managing these safety considerations, patients can effectively incorporate herbal remedies into their care plans while minimizing risks and maximizing therapeutic benefits.

IX

Other Key Approaches to Management

Alternative Therapies: In addition to conventional and herbal treatments, several alternative therapies may support the management of long COVID symptoms. These approaches can provide complementary benefits and enhance overall well-being.

Acupuncture: Acupuncture, a traditional Chinese medicine practice, involves inserting fine needles into specific points on the body to stimulate energy flow and promote healing. It is often used to manage pain, reduce inflammation, and support immune function. For long COVID patients, acupuncture may help alleviate symptoms such as fatigue, joint pain, and respiratory issues. Some studies suggest that acupuncture can improve quality of life and reduce symptom severity, although more research is needed to fully understand its effectiveness in treating long COVID.

Chiropractic Care: Chiropractic care focuses on diagnosing and treating musculoskeletal disorders, particularly those related to spinal alignment. Chiropractors use manual adjustments to correct misalignments and improve nerve function, which can help alleviate pain and improve mobility. For long COVID patients, chiropractic care may address musculoskeletal discomfort, such as back pain or joint stiffness, and support overall physical function. It is important to work with a qualified chiropractor to ensure that treatments are safe and appropriate for individual health needs.

Massage Therapy: Massage therapy involves manipulating soft tissues to relieve tension, improve circulation, and promote relaxation. Techniques such as deep tissue massage or myofascial release can help reduce muscle aches, joint pain, and stress associated with long COVID. Regular massage therapy may enhance recovery by improving blood flow, reducing inflammation, and supporting mental well-being. As with other therapies, it is important to consult with a licensed massage therapist and discuss any health concerns or contraindications.

Incorporating these alternative therapies into a comprehensive management plan can provide additional support and improve quality of life for long COVID patients, complementing conventional and herbal treatments.

Innovative Treatments

Hyperbaric Oxygen Therapy (HBOT): Hyperbaric Oxygen Therapy involves breathing pure oxygen in a pressurized room or chamber, which enhances oxygen delivery to tissues and promotes healing. For long COVID patients, HBOT may offer benefits by reducing inflammation, promoting tissue repair, and improving oxygenation in areas affected by the virus. Some preliminary studies suggest that HBOT could help alleviate symptoms such as fatigue, brain fog, and chronic pain. However, more research is needed to fully establish its efficacy and safety for long COVID, as it is currently used mainly for conditions like chronic wounds and decompression sickness.

Stem Cell Therapy: Stem cell therapy is an innovative treatment that involves using stem cells to repair or regenerate damaged tissues. For long COVID, this approach aims to address persistent inflammation and damage in various organs. Stem cells have the potential to modulate the immune response, reduce inflammation, and promote tissue repair. Clinical trials are exploring the effectiveness of stem cell therapy in treating long COVID-related conditions such as lung damage and cardiovascular issues. While promising, stem cell therapy remains experimental, and its use is subject to ongoing research and regulatory review to ensure safety and effectiveness.

Nutritional Genomics: Nutritional genomics, also known as nutrigenomics, studies the interaction between nutrition and genes to personalize dietary recommendations. For long COVID patients, this approach involves tailoring nutrition plans based on individual genetic profiles to optimize health and recovery. By understanding how specific nutrients affect gene expression and metabolic pathways, nutritional genomics can help address issues such as inflammation, immune function, and overall well-being. This innovative approach aims to provide personalized dietary strategies that enhance treatment outcomes and support long-term health.

These innovative treatments represent exciting developments in managing long COVID, offering new possibilities for improving patient outcomes through advanced and personalized approaches.

Lifestyle Modifications

Stress Management Techniques: Managing stress is crucial for long COVID patients, as chronic stress can exacerbate symptoms and hinder recovery. Techniques such as deep breathing exercises, progressive muscle relaxation, and mindfulness-based stress reduction can help lower stress levels and improve overall well-being. Cognitive-behavioral strategies, including setting realistic goals and developing coping mechanisms, also play a role in managing stress. Integrating these techniques into daily routines can help patients better handle the emotional and physical challenges associated with long COVID, potentially leading to improved symptom management and quality of life.

Mind-Body Practices (Yoga, Meditation): Mind-body practices like yoga and meditation are beneficial for long COVID patients, offering both physical and mental health benefits. Yoga combines physical postures, breathing exercises, and mindfulness to improve flexibility, strength, and relaxation. It can help alleviate musculoskeletal pain, enhance respiratory function, and reduce stress. Meditation, on the other hand, focuses on mindfulness and relaxation, which can help manage anxiety, improve mental clarity, and enhance emotional resilience. Regular practice of these techniques can support overall recovery by addressing both physical and psychological aspects of long COVID.

Environmental Modifications: Creating a supportive environment is essential for managing long COVID symptoms. This includes optimizing living spaces to reduce exposure to environmental stressors and improve comfort. For example, ensuring good air quality, reducing noise pollution, and creating a clutter-free, relaxing space can contribute to overall well-being. Ergonomic adjustments, such as using supportive furniture and organizing daily tasks to minimize physical strain, can also help manage symptoms like fatigue and musculoskeletal pain. By making these environmental modifications, patients can create a more conducive environment for healing and managing long COVID effectively.

Implementing these lifestyle modifications can play a significant role in supporting recovery and enhancing daily functioning for long COVID patients.

X

Living with Long COVID

Impact on Daily Life: Long COVID can profoundly affect daily life, altering routines and responsibilities. Persistent symptoms such as fatigue, brain fog, and physical discomfort often hinder one's ability to perform everyday tasks, impacting overall quality of life. Simple activities like household chores, shopping, or even social interactions can become overwhelming, leading to frustration and a sense of loss of independence.

Personal and Professional Challenges: The challenges extend to both personal and professional spheres. Personally, individuals may face difficulties maintaining relationships and fulfilling roles within the family due to ongoing health issues. Professionally, long COVID can impair job performance, leading to reduced productivity or even job loss. Adjustments in work schedules, responsibilities, or even career changes may be necessary to accommodate the limitations imposed by the condition. This can lead to financial stress and affect self-esteem.

Adapting to Limitations: Adapting to the limitations imposed by long COVID involves a process of acceptance and adjustment. It requires developing new strategies for managing daily activities, such as pacing oneself, prioritizing tasks, and seeking support from family, friends, or professional resources. Embracing these adaptations and seeking accommodations, whether through modified work arrangements or support services, can help individuals navigate the challenges of living with long COVID and maintain a sense of normalcy and well-being.

Quality of Life Considerations

Mental and Emotional Health: Long COVID can significantly impact mental and emotional health, contributing to feelings of anxiety, depression, and isolation. Persistent symptoms and the uncertainty of recovery may lead to stress and emotional distress. Addressing mental health is crucial for overall well-being. Engaging in therapeutic interventions such as counseling or cognitive-behavioral therapy can help manage symptoms and improve mental resilience. Regular self-care practices, including mindfulness and relaxation techniques, also play a vital role in supporting emotional health.

Social Support Networks: Social support is essential for maintaining quality of life when living with long COVID. A strong support network, including family, friends, and support groups, provides emotional comfort, practical assistance, and a sense of connection. Social interactions can help alleviate feelings of isolation and offer encouragement and understanding. Support groups, both in-person and online, provide a platform for sharing experiences and strategies, which can be empowering and validating. Building and maintaining these social connections can help individuals feel less alone and more supported in their journey through long COVID.

By addressing both mental health needs and fostering strong social connections, individuals can better manage the challenges of long COVID and enhance their overall quality of life.

Coping Mechanisms

Strategies for Resilience: Developing strategies for resilience is vital for managing the ongoing challenges of long COVID. Techniques such as setting realistic goals, practicing self-compassion, and maintaining a flexible mindset can enhance emotional strength.

Establishing a daily routine that includes time for rest and self-care helps manage symptoms and fosters a sense of normalcy. Engaging in regular physical activity, even at a low intensity, and practicing stress-relief techniques like mindfulness or meditation can support overall well-being. Building a support network of friends, family, and healthcare providers also provides practical and emotional support, aiding in the adaptation to the condition.

Finding Meaning and Purpose: Finding meaning and purpose in the midst of long COVID can significantly improve mental health and coping. Reflecting on personal values and setting meaningful goals can provide motivation and a sense of direction. Engaging in activities that bring joy or fulfillment, such as hobbies, volunteer work, or creative pursuits, helps create a positive focus and counteracts feelings of loss or frustration. Many individuals find purpose through connecting with others who share similar experiences, participating in advocacy, or contributing to long COVID research. By identifying and pursuing sources of meaning, individuals can navigate the challenges of long COVID with greater resilience and a renewed sense of purpose.

XI

Research and Future Directions

Current Research Efforts: The field of long COVID research is rapidly evolving as scientists work to better understand the condition and develop effective treatments. Major studies are investigating various aspects of long COVID, including its underlying mechanisms, symptom profiles, and potential therapeutic interventions. Research efforts focus on identifying biomarkers, understanding the impact on different organ systems, and exploring the effectiveness of various treatment modalities.

Major Studies and Initiatives: Significant studies and initiatives are shaping the current landscape of long COVID research. For example, the National Institutes of Health (NIH) launched the RECOVER Initiative, a large-scale research program aimed at understanding long COVID and developing strategies to improve patient outcomes. Similarly, the UK-based Study of Long COVID (PHOSP-COVID) investigates the long-term effects of COVID-19 in hospitalized patients, providing valuable insights into symptom persistence and recovery trajectories. These initiatives are crucial for identifying effective treatments and informing public health strategies.

Research Institutions and Collaborations: Leading research institutions and collaborative networks are at the forefront of long COVID research. Institutions such as Johns Hopkins University, the Mayo Clinic, and the University College London are conducting extensive studies on long COVID and contributing to the global knowledge base. Collaborative efforts, including international partnerships and multidisciplinary research teams, are essential for advancing understanding and developing comprehensive management strategies. By pooling resources and expertise, these collaborations enhance the ability to address the complexities of long COVID and work towards effective solutions for affected individuals.

Ongoing research and collaboration are critical for advancing the understanding of long COVID, improving patient care, and developing innovative treatments to address this evolving health challenge.

Knowledge Gaps and Challenges

Unanswered Questions: Despite significant research into long COVID, several unanswered questions remain. Key areas of uncertainty include the precise mechanisms underlying persistent symptoms and why some individuals develop long COVID while others do not. Understanding the role of viral persistence, immune system dysregulation, and genetic factors is crucial for developing targeted treatments. Additionally, the variability in symptom presentation and recovery trajectories raises questions about effective management strategies and individualized care. Research must continue to address these gaps to provide clearer answers and better support for those affected.

Methodological Issues: Methodological challenges also pose obstacles in long COVID research. Variability in study designs, definitions of long COVID, and outcome measures can complicate the comparison of results across different studies. Small sample sizes, short follow-up periods, and lack of standardization in diagnostic criteria further impact the reliability and generalizability of findings. Additionally, capturing the full range of symptoms and their impact on quality of life requires comprehensive and longitudinal studies. Addressing these methodological issues is essential for obtaining robust data and developing effective interventions. Improved research design, standardized protocols, and larger, well-characterized cohorts are needed to overcome these challenges and advance our understanding of long COVID.

Future Directions

Promising Areas of Research: Several promising areas of research are emerging in the field of long COVID. One key focus is identifying specific biomarkers that can predict and diagnose long COVID more accurately. By understanding the biological markers associated with persistent symptoms, researchers aim to develop targeted therapies and personalized treatment plans. Another promising area is the investigation of novel antiviral and anti-inflammatory treatments that could address the underlying causes of long COVID. Research into the role of gut microbiota and its impact on long COVID symptoms is also gaining traction, potentially revealing new avenues for intervention.

Potential Breakthroughs: Potential breakthroughs in long COVID research include advancements in precision medicine and regenerative therapies. Precision medicine approaches, which tailor treatments based on individual genetic and biochemical profiles, could lead to more effective management strategies. Stem cell therapy and other regenerative treatments hold promise for repairing tissue damage and modulating immune responses in long COVID patients. Additionally, innovations in digital health technologies, such as wearable devices and mobile health apps, could enhance symptom monitoring and management, providing real-time data to inform treatment decisions. As research progresses, these advancements have the potential to significantly improve outcomes for individuals living with long COVID, offering hope for more effective and personalized approaches to care.

XII

Resources for Patients

Websites and Organizations: Several reputable websites and organizations provide valuable information and support for individuals with long COVID. The Centers for Disease Control and Prevention (CDC) offers comprehensive resources on long COVID, including symptom guides, management strategies, and research updates. The National Institutes of Health (NIH) also provides insights into ongoing research and clinical trials related to long COVID. Additionally, organizations such as the Long COVID Alliance and the Body Politic Long COVID Support Group offer resources tailored to long COVID patients, including educational materials, advocacy information, and community support. These websites and organizations are vital for staying informed about the latest developments, accessing self-care strategies, and connecting with support networks.

Long COVID Clinics and Support Groups: Specialized long COVID clinics provide multidisciplinary care tailored to the complex needs of long COVID patients. These clinics often include experts in fields such as pulmonology, cardiology, neurology, and rehabilitation, offering comprehensive assessments and personalized treatment plans. For example, the Post COVID-19 Recovery Clinic at Mount Sinai Health System and similar centers in various regions are dedicated to evaluating and managing long COVID symptoms. Support groups, both in-person and online, play a crucial role in connecting patients with others who share similar experiences. Platforms like Facebook groups, Reddit communities, and specialized forums offer spaces for individuals to share coping strategies, seek advice, and find emotional support. Engaging with these resources can provide practical assistance and a sense of community for those navigating the challenges of long COVID.

Resources for Healthcare Providers

Training and Education Materials: Healthcare providers can access various training and education materials to enhance their understanding of long COVID and improve patient care. Professional organizations such as the American Thoracic Society and the European Respiratory Society offer webinars, continuing medical education (CME) courses, and workshops focused on long COVID. These resources provide up-to-date information on symptom management, diagnostic approaches, and treatment options. Additionally, specialized training programs are available through institutions like the Mayo Clinic and Johns Hopkins University, offering detailed insights into the latest research and clinical practices.

Guidelines and Best Practices: Comprehensive guidelines and best practices for managing long COVID are provided by several authoritative sources. The National Institute for Health and Care Excellence (NICE) and the World Health Organization (WHO) have published guidelines outlining diagnostic criteria, management strategies, and recommended treatments for long COVID. These guidelines are designed to help healthcare providers standardize care and ensure evidence-based practices. Additionally, the American College of Physicians and similar organizations offer clinical practice guidelines and resources for developing individualized patient management plans. By utilizing these guidelines and staying updated with the latest research, healthcare providers can enhance their approach to long COVID, improving patient outcomes and supporting effective management of this complex condition.

Advocacy and Policy

Patient Advocacy Groups: Patient advocacy groups play a crucial role in raising awareness and driving action for long COVID. Organizations such as the Long COVID Alliance and Body Politic work to amplify the voices of those affected by long COVID, advocating for better research funding, improved healthcare access, and patient rights. These groups often engage in lobbying efforts to influence policy changes, support legislative initiatives, and collaborate with healthcare providers to address gaps in care. By mobilizing patient communities and collaborating with stakeholders, advocacy groups help ensure that long COVID receives the attention and resources it needs.

Public Health Policies and Initiatives: Public health policies and initiatives are essential for addressing long COVID on a broader scale. Governments and health organizations are increasingly recognizing the need for comprehensive strategies to manage and mitigate long COVID's impact. Initiatives may include funding for research, development of clinical guidelines, and creation of long COVID clinics. For example, the U.S. government's RECOVER Initiative aims to study and address long COVID, while the UK's NHS has established post-COVID-19 services to provide specialized care.

These policies help shape the response to long COVID, ensuring that it is addressed in public health planning and resource allocation, and guiding healthcare systems in delivering effective care to affected individuals.

Conclusion

Summary of Key Points

This book has explored the multifaceted nature of long COVID, from its definition and causes to its wide-ranging impacts on health and daily life. We've examined the theories behind long COVID, including viral persistence, immune system dysregulation, and autonomic nervous system involvement. The symptoms and their variability were discussed, highlighting the challenge of diagnosing and managing this complex condition. We covered medical and alternative treatments, emphasizing the importance of a comprehensive approach that includes physical rehabilitation, mental health support, and dietary strategies. The role of herbal remedies, innovative treatments, and lifestyle modifications were also addressed as part of a holistic management plan. Finally, we reviewed the current research landscape, identified knowledge gaps, and explored the resources available for both patients and healthcare providers.

Final Thoughts and Encouragement: Living with long COVID can be challenging, but with the right resources and support, individuals can navigate these difficulties and work towards recovery. It is essential to maintain hope and seek out comprehensive care that addresses both physical and emotional well-being. Engaging with support networks and utilizing available resources can significantly enhance the quality of life for those affected.

Call to Action for Research and Support: Continued research and advocacy are crucial for improving our understanding of long COVID and developing effective treatments. Support for ongoing research initiatives and patient advocacy efforts is needed to drive progress and ensure that those affected by long COVID receive the care and attention they deserve. By working together—patients, healthcare providers, and researchers—we can advance our knowledge and improve outcomes for all individuals impacted by this condition.